LIVER DETOX
Energize Your Life

Rhody Lake

live
hea|thy
now!

HEALTHY LIVING PUBLICATIONS
Summertown, Tennessee

Cover and interior design: Scattaregia Design

Healthy Living Publications,
a division of Book Publishing Company
PO Box 99
Summertown, TN 38483
888-260-8458
bookpubco.com

ISBN: 978-1-57067-350-4

> **Disclaimer**
> The information in this book is presented for educational purposes only. It isn't intended to be a substitute for the medical advice of a physician, dietitian, or other healthcare professional.

Printed in the United States of America

21 20 19 18 17   1 2 3 4 5 6 7 8 9

Library of Congress Cataloging-in-Publication Data

Names: Lake, Rhody, author.
Title: Liver detox : energize your life / Rhody Lake.
Description: Summertown, Tennessee : Healthy Living Publications, [2017]
Identifiers: LCCN 2017018680 (print) | LCCN 2017015204 (ebook) | ISBN
  9781570678493 (E-book) | ISBN 9781570673504 (paperback)
Subjects: LCSH: Detoxification (Health) | Detoxification (Health)--Recipes. |
  Self-care, Health--Popular works.
Classification: LCC RA784.5 (print) | LCC RA784.5 .L35 2017 (ebook) | DDC 613--dc23
LC record available at https://lccn.loc.gov/2017018680

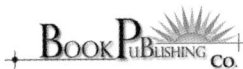

BOOK PUBLISHING CO.

We chose to print this title on responsibly harvested paper stock certified by the Forest Stewardship Council®, an independent auditor of responsible forestry practices. For more information, visit https://us.fsc.org.

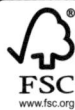

FSC
www.fsc.org

MIX
Paper from
responsible sources
FSC® C005010

CONTENTS

Introduction

All the organs, glands, muscles, and tissues of the body function in unison to make a harmonious and homogeneous whole, but the liver plays perhaps the most important role. Indeed, "liver" comes from the old English word for "life." Keeping your liver happy is essential to your life, so it's truly worthwhile to find out how to treat what the Chinese call "the father of all organs." Perhaps we should adopt this common Russian greeting: How's your liver today?

You may be taking treatments for any number of health problems— allergies, asthma, constipation, diabetes, high cholesterol, irritable bowel syndrome, or skin rashes—not knowing that the real problem stems from your liver. This large and very important detoxifying organ could be clogged, sluggish, ailing, and unhappy—in short, dysfunctional. Ultimately, this may all be the result of poor diet and lifestyle. Liver toxins can be found in almost all the foods most people have been raised on.

The good news is that the liver is very forgiving. Optimum liver function can be restored, and even a damaged liver can be regenerated. It's all a matter of knowing what to do and what not to do. The purpose of this book is to motivate you to consider your liver and adopt a dietary protocol that will allow it to detoxify daily. You're the only one responsible for choosing what you put into your body. When you assist your liver with doing its job well, you will function better on all cylinders—mentally, emotionally, and physically.

A Toxic World

The liver works as part of a team in your body, and its job is to detoxify. The need to detoxify is more important than ever before because we live in a toxic world, largely as a result of so-called advances from the industrial revolution: agricultural chemicals used in farming, chemical food additives, pharmaceutical drugs, chlorination and fluoridation of water, car exhaust, and indoor pollutants from chemical cleaners, paints, carpeting, and furniture. All these substances contribute to a toxic environment and burden the body's coping mechanisms.

But the greatest assault on the body, and the liver in particular, is from modern food. Denatured, processed foods, loaded with chemical additives, are unique to the last hundred years and cause greater stress on the liver than our ancestors experienced. The liver must work constantly to eliminate these toxins through the bowels, kidneys, lungs, and skin so they don't get into the bloodstream. An overload of toxins means all the other organs are overloaded too, and each must do more than it can adequately handle. As a result, we experience symptoms that physicians associate with disease. Unfortunately, doctors often treat just these symptoms and never investigate the root cause.

Among the most insidious of these toxins are the trans-fatty acids found in hydrogenated oils, which have been used in many processed or packaged food items. These oils, artificially hardened by metal and hydrogen gas, produce fatty acid trans isomers, which are not natural to the human body. Because trans isomers are foreign, our bodies don't know what to do with them. Eating processed, hydrogenated, man-made fats puts us at greater risk of breast cancer, diabetes, and heart disease than eating animal fats. Fortunately, the consumption of trans fats has sharply declined since 2006, when the US Food and Drug Administration required that trans-fat content be included on food labels. In the near future, these fats will most likely be banned except in rare instances.

Even though the use of trans fats has fallen out of favor, food manufacturers continue to experiment with other substances that mimic the fats that make foods so palatable and appealing. Olestra, also known by the brand name Olean, is an example of an artificial fat that was designed to go through the digestive system without being absorbed. It's been reported to cause severe intestinal cramps, diarrhea, and other side effects. The liver is severely compromised when it must dispose of such toxins.

Ultimately, what's required for optimal health is a new eating pattern and a liver-cleansing diet that will enable all the assisting organs—the bowels, intestines, kidneys, and pancreas—to function at their best. When such a diet is adopted, the liver never becomes blocked with toxic waste. When the liver processes natural fats, it manufactures normal amounts of cholesterol and assists in the production of bile. As a result, you'll be the picture of health.

The Body's Pathways of Detoxification

You have only one liver, so you must keep it functioning well in order for your body to properly detoxify. Since only the liver can purify the bloodstream, it's crucial that you keep it happy and cleanse it regularly by eating a daily regimen of specific foods and nutrients. Toxins will then be easily excreted through prescribed pathways—from the gallbladder to bile to the bowels, and from the kidneys to the bladder.

Via these pathways, we eliminate alcohol, food additives, insecticides, microorganisms (parasites), pharmaceutical drugs, and other toxins. When these pathways are clogged or overloaded, toxins must then be eliminated through the skin, resulting in acne blemishes, brown spots, eczema, facial flushing, itchy rashes, and rosacea.

Bile Balance

Bile is an essential player in the digestive process. It's a bitter, yellow-green fluid that's produced by the liver and stored in the gallbladder, where it's released as needed for digestion. Bile breaks down fat into small globules and assists in absorbing fats and fat-soluble vitamins (A, D, E, and K). It also helps convert beta-carotene into vitamin A and frees the small intestine of potentially harmful microorganisms. Finally, bile promotes peristalsis (movement) in the bowels to keep the feces moving along the digestive tract and out of the body as waste, thereby preventing constipation, the bane of Western civilization.

Barring overindulgence, the liver should be able to produce the bile necessary for digestion and elimination, keeping all the other pathways clear. However, modern food manufacturers have developed chemical additives and preservatives that only have recently pervaded our food supply. The liver treats these unrecognizable substances as toxins. If there are too many of these toxins to remove through the normal digestive process, the body will attempt to eliminate them through the skin. A toxic overload of artificially hardened fats and other manufactured food substances will eventually result in degeneration and disease.

Your Liver or Your Life

The liver is designed to operate with clocklike precision. At about two o'clock in the morning, it begins to process the nutrients from the evening meal. If that meal was light and not eaten too late in the day, the liver can easily manage it, sending sufficient bile to the gallbladder for the next stage of digestion. If you eat a heavy meal and have it late in the evening, the liver needs to work overtime—until about eight o'clock in the morning or later. The consequence of a sluggish liver is early morning fatigue. You'll want to stay under the covers and complain that you're not a "morning person." In reality, it's your liver that is struggling that time of day—it hasn't been able to get rid of its toxic load.

Waking exhausted, you try to jump-start the day with a cup of coffee, but the caffeine compromises your liver even more. You may choose to treat yourself to a bagel and cream cheese for breakfast, more coffee midmorning, and French fries with pizza for lunch. The liver's response to this toxic overload of caffeine, sugar, and fat is to work at a frantic pace. If your regular diet also includes packaged bread, chips, cookies, crackers, dips, and spreads full of chemical additives, your liver will have more to process than it can handle, and disease will be the result.

Liver Distress Signals

When you feel fatigued, listless, and at odds with the world, more than likely your liver is experiencing toxic distress. Even young people can have a clogged and toxin-loaded liver, which does not bode well for their future health. If their diet regularly includes the processed foods that abound in fast-food restaurants and vending machines, they can expect an ongoing series of symptoms that medical doctors will tend to treat with prescription drugs (contributing even more to the body's toxic load), not recognizing the underlying cause—a miserable liver. The following are some of the signals of liver distress:

- abdominal bloating
- acne blemishes
- acne rosacea
- brown spots (liver spots) on the skin
- cellulite
- chronic fatigue syndrome
- compromised pancreas
- depression
- eczema
- elevated cholesterol

- high blood pressure
- hot flashes
- indigestion
- irritability
- irritable bowel
  syndrome (IBS)
- pimples
- pot belly
- weight gain

Most people treat these symptoms with over-the-counter or prescription drugs and carry on unaware that their lifestyle is destroying their liver. If you've decided to change course and be responsible for your health, this book will give you the information you need to improve the state of your liver and achieve better health.

Easing the Digestion Process

Many people have misconceptions about what constitutes a healthy diet, which is the cornerstone to good digestion. The first step toward improved health is knowing what you should eat: fresh, whole fruits and vegetables, eaten raw or cooked as lightly as possible; cooked grains and legumes; fresh, raw nuts and seeds; and whole-grain breads and cereals. These are the types of foods our ancestors ate.

If you purchase any packaged foods, take the time to read the list of ingredients. If they're numerous, mysterious, or difficult to pronounce (such as acetic anhydride, ammonium hydroxide, calcium aluminum silicate, sodium hypochlorite, or magnesium stearate), put the item back on the shelf and walk to the produce aisle instead.

Digestion begins in the mouth, and food should be well pulverized and salivated through chewing. Although daily intake of water (eight glasses a day) is essential, avoid drinking water with meals. Consuming liquids with meals dilutes the stomach's hydrochloric acid, which breaks down food for proper digestion, destroys any bacteria in the food, and facilitates rapid bowel function. When there's adequate hydrochloric acid in the stomach, vitamins and minerals are properly utilized; but when hydrochloric acid is diluted or insufficient, food putrefies, causing gas, bloating, and discomfort. In addition, the liver will be stymied and won't be able to do its job. As a general rule, drink water two hours after a meal or half an hour before meals.

Aging and Hydrochloric Acid Deficiencies

Older people are almost always lacking in hydrochloric acid. Deficiencies often show up in people forty years of age and up, but even teenagers can have deficiencies as a result of poor diet.

Bulk Up Your Diet

Fiber in the diet is essential for the liver to function well. Fiber is the garbage truck that carries away cholesterol. Refined grains have had this important component removed, and foods made from refined grains—such as white bread, pastas, and many breakfast cereals—are no longer good sources of fiber. To get a better handle on your cholesterol levels, adopt a daily dietary regimen of whole foods, such as cooked intact grains, fresh fruits, legumes, raw or steamed vegetables, and whole-grain bread. Emphasize raw foods— up to 75 percent of your diet if possible. Eating whole and especially raw foods will give you sufficient fiber to facilitate the peristaltic movement of the bowels.

Peristalsis is a series of muscle contractions that move food and waste along the intestinal tract. Fiber soaks up water at ten to thirty times its weight, so you'll need to consume lots of water for proper elimination. Digestion is impeded when either too little water or fiber is consumed throughout the day.

When you're healthy, your organs work in harmony during every bodily process. Every function is important and affects every other function. When you simply drink water and do not consume fiber-rich foods, the water will be expelled through the urinary tract without removing any toxins. Faulty elimination of toxins hampers the bile duct and pancreatic ducts and engorges the liver. The poor pancreas can't supply sufficient digestive enzymes to the small intestine so the body can digest food. And when digestion stops, so does the proper assimilation of nutrients.

Fiber Supplements

If you're having trouble with elimination, a fiber supplement that includes psyllium husks will add necessary bulk. Be sure to take adequate amounts of water along with it—water is required to ensure the psyllium husks swell up and then move out.

Weight Loss

The liver is a fat-burning machine, and it's instrumental for normalizing weight by pumping excess fat out of the body through bile and into the small intestine. Eating a diet high in fiber reduces the recirculation of fats and other toxins from the gut to the liver. When you eat a low-fiber diet, the bad fats, especially trans fats and cholesterol, get into the bloodstream. In addition, an adequate amount of high-density lipoproteins, known as HDL cholesterol (the good kind), isn't manufactured, and low-density lipoproteins, known as LDL cholesterol (the bad kind), attach to blood vessel walls.

The good fats are found in freshly pressed oils derived from seeds and nuts, such as flaxseeds, pumpkin seeds, sunflower seeds, and walnuts. They provide essential omega-3 and omega-6 fatty acids, which the body can't manufacture. These important oils are easily processed by the liver and help the body maintain a healthy weight. (For more information about essential fats, read *Good Fats and Oils* by Siegfried Gursche.)

A roll of fat at the waistline of either men or women can be a sign of what is commonly called a fatty liver. This refers to a liver that has stopped processing fat and instead has become a fat-storing organ, engorged and swollen with greasy deposits. No matter how much people exercise, they won't be able to remove this fat roll unless their liver function improves. Eliminating this excess fat requires a protocol of detoxification, followed by a liver-cleansing regimen. This will take both time and patience. Liver restoration won't happen overnight and could take three to five months or longer. Once the accumulated fat is removed, however, weight loss will occur, vitality will improve, and "liverish" symptoms will disappear.

Parasites and Poor Elimination

Parasites are yet another potential problem caused by improper elimination. A toxic buildup in the bowel creates an environment conducive to parasites. Parasite incubation time is quick—about thirty-six hours. If you haven't had a bowel movement for several days, you're increasing the chance of parasites moving in.

Kitchen Wisdom: Foods to Choose

Fortunately, you don't have to go any farther than your own kitchen to begin detoxifying and improving your liver function. It all starts with what you choose to eat. Adopting a liver-cleansing diet is relatively easy and painless. It just takes awareness and the will to shift your diet to include foods that are life promoting and liver enhancing. Food really is your best medicine. Choose foods that are natural, whole, and unprocessed, just as nature made them, as these are the ones your digestive system and cleansing organs can metabolize most effectively. Efficient metabolism equates to good health.

In order for the body to properly fulfill the process of liver detoxification, the following nutrients are required:
- amino acids (cysteine, glycine, glutamine, taurine)
- antioxidants (carotenoids, vitamins E and C, and sulfured phytochemicals in foods such as cruciferous vegetables and garlic)
- folic acid and other B vitamins
- glutathione

Vegetables and Fruits

Raw vegetables and fruits are rich both in fiber and water content and are the foundation of sound eating habits. Choose brightly colored foods, such as dark green leafy vegetables, tomatoes, red and green peppers, orange fruits and veggies (such as carrots, papayas, squash, and yams), red cabbage, purple beets and eggplant, and juicy oranges.

These vibrant, rich colors aren't there by accident. Not only do these hues make nutritious foods attractive, but they're also a sign that the foods contain powerful antioxidants and carotenoids, which are essential substances for high-performance metabolism and optimum liver function. For instance, tomatoes contain lycopene, an antioxidant considered the most powerful of all the dietary carotenoids. Carrots provide beta-carotene, and beets offer the antioxidant anthocyanin.

If you eat these vegetables in the form of freshly pressed juices, your body will quickly absorb the nutrients without requiring a lengthy digestion time. (For more information, read *Juicing for the Health of It!* by Siegfried Gursche.) Freshly pressed vegetable juice is the best liver-cleansing food and should be part of the daily diet.

Eating whole, raw fruits and vegetables, either fresh or juiced, provides the body with a number of vitamins, phytochemicals, and other nutrients that are destroyed when foods are cooked. When you do cook vegetables, lightly steam them to preserve as many nutrients as possible, and never overcook them.

Fats and Oils

Freshly pressed oils, such as flaxseed oil, olive oil, sesame oil, and sunflower oil, are easily emulsified and digested and are essential to building healthy membranes around the liver's cells. However, fresh seed and nut oils are easily damaged by light and heat. Buy them only if they are unrefined and stored in dark glass bottles. Be sure to read the pressing date on the bottle's label to determine the oil's freshness. Flaxseed oil is especially delicate and should only be purchased from merchants who keep the oil refrigerated. Freshly pressed nut and seed oils can go rancid in a few weeks—and rancid oils are carcinogenic, resulting in more toxins for the liver to cope with.

Refined oils have a much longer shelf life than unrefined oils, which makes them easy to transport over long distances. However, the high temperature used in the refining process changes the molecular structure of these oils and creates the trans-fatty acids the liver must avoid. If you want to live a long life, eliminate these oils from your diet.

Instead of margarine, use drops of fresh, unrefined oils on breads, cooked whole grains, and vegetables. Do as the Italians do and dip slices of whole-grain bread in extra-virgin olive oil that's been seasoned with cracked black pepper and a few grains of sea salt.

Fresh raw nuts and seeds are natural protein sources the body can easily assimilate and digest. Nature wraps them in a protective coating containing enzyme inhibitors, known as phytates, that keep them from rotting and prevent their oil from going rancid. (Unshelled nuts and seeds will keep for years as long as they're kept dry.) Although phytates have a few protective qualities for people, as they lower cholesterol and may protect against some cancers, these enzyme inhibitors are difficult for humans to digest. However, soaking and juicing help break down the phytates, and those processes also release calcium, iron, and other minerals that would otherwise be bound to these foods. Therefore, nuts and seeds should be soaked in water and drained before they're eaten. (Grains and legumes also have enzyme inhibitors, and that's why it's important to always soak dried beans, lentils, and peas before cooking them, and to always discard the soak water.)

Soy or No Soy?

Whole soybeans are a good source of oil as well as protein. However, all soybean oil has been refined and heat processed. It's not a natural product, even if it's labeled as "natural." Soy products present other problems as well. The soybeans used in many processed food products are not the same beans that Asians have been eating for generations. Soybean crops in North America and elsewhere around the world are big business, and the beans grown by commercial farmers have been hybridized for decades as a normal aspect of plant science. Add to this the present practice of altering the bean's intrinsic genes. The result is that almost all soybeans currently grown are genetically engineered, and no one knows the cumulative effects this will have on human health. Genetically altered food products have not been proven safe and no long-term tests have been done on how they affect us. The best way to protect yourself and your family is to purchase only certified organic soy foods, including tofu, tempeh, and naturally fermented tamari. Look for certification on the package label.

Great Grains

Whole grains can be part of the happy-liver diet, but for some people the gluten found in wheat and a handful of other grains can present problems. Whole wheat bread, crackers, and other baked goods may be relatively easy for you to metabolize if your ancestors traditionally incorporated these foods in their diets. People whose ancestors did not consume wheat (such as indigenous American cultures and the rural Chinese) can have difficulty digesting gluten, the primary protein found in wheat. Most whole grains can be beneficial in a liver-cleansing diet for individuals who have no trouble digesting them.

Good, Clean Water

Water helps all the internal organs operate at their best, and it's essential for a happy liver. To be an effective hydrating and cleansing agent, water should be made up of molecules that are configured much like snowflakes—with no other substances included. Unfortunately, this kind of water is only obtainable in remote, pristine areas of the world, and it definitely does not come out of city water pipes.

Tap water is chlorinated and may also be fluoridated. Both chlorine and fluoride are toxic substances the liver must deal with. Don't add them to your liver load! Purchase steam-distilled water for drinking, outfit your kitchen tap with a water filter, or use a home distiller to reclaim the life-giving properties of the water from your public water system or private well.

Foods to Refuse

A liver-cleansing diet basically involves eating with common sense. Unfortunately, modern food processing and marketing easily distract us from making commonsense decisions about which foods are appealing and nutritious. Manufacturing foods with cheap ingredients enhanced by chemical additives that make them practically addictive is how the food industry rakes in money. It takes a conscious effort to avoid these tempting foods and choose whole, natural ingredients instead.

Nonfood Ingredients

The list of items to avoid includes all the processed and packaged foods produced by the giant food manufacturers. These so-called foods, loaded with nonfood ingredients, have become the mainstay of food producers at the expense of human health. Avoid artificial sweeteners, caffeine, chemical food colors, flavor enhancers, heat-damaged fats, hydrogenated oils, pesticides, preservatives, sugar in all its forms, and the many other nonfood additives listed on food labels. All of these are liver toxins. When these poisons are ingested, your busy liver becomes overwhelmed trying to filter them out so they don't get into your bloodstream. Enjoy a wholesome, wholefoods diet and relieve your liver of all that extra work!

Sweet Treats

Use natural sweeteners, such as dried fruit, honey, and maple syrup, only in moderation. Sweeteners are not part of the regular happy-liver diet no matter how much they tempt your taste buds, and refined sugar is the most detrimental. Most people consume far too much sugar in their diets. You'll go a long way toward keeping your liver happy and healthy if you learn to live without sweet foods. If you make a habit of leaving out sugar when you're preparing food, even when a recipe calls for it, your taste buds will eventually adapt for the better.

Probiotics

Increasingly, health researchers are discovering that our physical well-being relies in great part on the millions of friendly bacteria found in the human digestive system. These friendly organisms help fight harmful bacteria, promote the absorption of nutrients, break down fiber in the large intestine, protect against food allergies, and boost the immune system. But healthy gut flora can be compromised by a diet that's consistently high in fat and low in fiber, potentially leading to allergies (including increased sensitivity to pollen), candidiasis (an overgrowth of *Candida albicans*), chronic inflammation, overweight, and skin problems.

Probiotics work to restore the balance of bacteria in the intestinal tract by increasing or replacing these friendly organisms. A number of fermented foods, such as kombucha, miso, unprocessed sauerkraut and pickles, and yogurt, are naturally rich in probiotics and have long played an important role in many traditional diets. Probiotics are also present in some cheeses, but this is becoming less prevalent with the mass production of dairy products. In addition, the incidence of dairy allergies and sensitivities has steadily been on the upswing, and all animal-based foods are coming under increased scrutiny because of their adverse effects on the environment. Choose plant-based fermented foods instead.

If you're struggling with health problems, consider taking a concentrated probiotic supplement, preferably the strongest formulation you can find. Blends with concentrations of fifty billion or more colony-forming units (CFUs) are worth the extra cost. Although gas and bloating are uncommon side effects of probiotics, if you experience any discomfort, just take a smaller amount. Lower concentrations are also fine as maintenance doses. Since probiotics are sensitive to heat, buy them from reputable retailers who keep them refrigerated, and store them in the refrigerator once you get them home.

Attitude Is Altitude

Consider the liver-cleansing diet as an adventure. Embarking on such a diet is like climbing a mountain to see the view from the top—a struggle, but worth the gain in altitude. You'll need to plan carefully, but most important of all, go forward with confidence and a positive mind-set. An upbeat attitude is very important for a healthy liver because the liver treats negative emotions, such as frustration, anger, and hostility, as toxins. The liver has difficulty processing these emotional toxins, so they get stored in the muscles and tissues of the body. The result is distress and disease.

E. E. Rogers, MD, a medical maverick who advocated the principles of nutritional healing over sixty years ago, said, "If you are intelligent enough to eat properly, it is better to also like it when you are doing it. The diet will work better if you do the necessary things in the proper spirit."

Be positive and grateful for what you have, and enjoy real food. Then your liver will relax and do its job properly.

The Liver Cleanse

A liver-cleansing procedure is sometimes called a liver flush. It's designed to cleanse the liver of toxins, fat, and sludge and to flush out the fatty and calcified deposits called gallstones. The longer that bile remains in the gall-bladder, the thicker this bitter, greenish liquid becomes and the greater the likelihood of stones forming. These stones also form when too little bile is produced. They in turn decrease the ability of the liver to make bile, resulting in less cholesterol and toxins being removed from the body.

Essential fatty acids from sources such as flaxseed oil and evening primrose oil stimulate bile production and help transport cholesterol and fatty sludge out of the liver. When we get rid of gallstones, our digestion improves dramatically, allergies cease to exist, and back pain disappears. It seems like a miracle—but it's not. It's just a greatly relieved liver that is now able to move toxins out. I don't recommend jumping into a liver flush unless you've been on the liver-cleansing diet for at least a few weeks. Ideally, the liver flush itself requires dietary preparation for one to two days in advance: eat only raw foods and drink eight to ten glasses of freshly pressed vegetable

juice and at least eight glasses of water daily. This cleansing regimen facilitates the process and lessens the chance of a bad reaction, such as nausea
or vomiting. If you're anxious about doing it, you probably shouldn't. Again,
attitude and confidence are important.

Perform the liver flush on a weekend, when you have the time to stick
to the protocol and rest, and also have ready access to a bathroom. Get up
bright and early, go for a long walk, and do deep-breathing exercises to
oxygenate the tissues, relax, and ease away any tension. Continue to drink
water throughout the day.

There are many recipes for flushing the liver and gallbladder. Any
regimen that makes use of the cleansing properties of cayenne, garlic,
lemon, and olive oil should work fairly well. The following is one method
I've found to be successful when I faithfully adhere to the protocol.

Squeeze enough grapefruit, lemons, or limes to make 11 ounces of
juice. Dilute the juice with 7 ounces of steam-distilled water (filtered water
will also do). Chop 1 to 2 cloves of fresh garlic and ½ teaspoon of fresh
gingerroot, then press both together in a garlic press to release their juices.
You can also use ½ teaspoon of cayenne instead of the ginger. Add the
garlic and ginger juice to the diluted fruit juice.

Pour 11 ounces of extra-virgin olive oil into a warm glass. The procedure is to swallow 3 tablespoons of the juice mixture and 3 tablespoons of
the olive oil every 15 minutes, relaxing between doses by lying down with
a hot water bottle over the liver area. This moist heat dilates the bile ducts
and helps to release small stones and sludge from the gallbladder. You
could also sit in a warm bath, but I find using a hot water bottle easier to do.

This recipe will leave you with some extra juice for sipping later. The juice itself is always beneficial as a cleansing morning drink.

The whole process can take several hours, so turn off your electronic devices and be patient. Enjoy the fact that you're doing something wonderful for your liver and thus your whole body. Bowel elimination will start to happen along with some possible discomfort and cramping. Don't be concerned about this. Massage your abdomen, following up the ascending colon, across the abdomen in line with the transverse colon, and down the descending colon. Sip fresh water, breathe deeply, and relax if you feel nauseous.

If you're stouthearted and curious, you can empty your bowels into a bedpan or commode chair in order to count the small greenish stones or grit that you pass with every movement. Some of them may be no bigger than a small pea; others may be large and soft, full of fatty sludge (cholesterol). Be happy that you're getting rid of them. And if you stay on a liver-cleansing diet, you may not produce any more. A healthy liver manufactures and secretes healthy bile, which prevents gallbladder inflammation and the formation of stones.

The day after the flush, stay on your liver-cleansing diet of freshly pressed vegetable juice, raw fruit and vegetables, and steamed and baked vegetables. Eat moderately and exercise.

Liver-Loving Herbs

The liver loves anything bitter. People around the world have long used bitter herbs for liver cleansing, especially after a grueling winter. Wild herbs, such as artichoke, dandelion greens, endive, garlic, lettuce, radicchio, and onion, were commonly harvested and dried for later use. All bitter herbs aid liver function and encourage the secretion of bile. Unfortunately, most varieties of cultivated herbs have had the bitter characteristics bred out of them through hybridizing. The popular iceberg lettuce, for instance, is essentially devoid of nutrients, but it has a long shelf life. Because of modern food marketing and distribution tactics, Western cultures have learned to like iceberg lettuce and hate bitters. But our bodies need bitters, and herbs are now the best sources of them.

Medicinal Herbs

Herbs that are specifically helpful for cleansing the liver include celandine, goldenseal, milk thistle, rue, and wormwood. Herbs are synergistic, which means they help each other to function. Medicinal herbs are best taken in compatible combinations and only for limited periods of time. Adhere to a protocol of three to six weeks, or vary your combinations daily, according to your needs.

Herbs can be taken in capsule form or as tea infusions that can be sipped throughout the day. The age-old recipe for Swedish bitters is a combination of eleven herbs that has been used effectively for hundreds of years. It's available at natural food stores as a packaged blend, but you can purchase the individual dried herbs, combine them yourself, and brew your own Swedish bitters tea, if you prefer.

Make an infusion by pouring boiling water over the leaves and blossoms and steeping them for five minutes or longer before straining and drinking. Berries can be steeped the same way, but roots and bark should be simmered for five to fifteen minutes to release their active ingredients. When using a combination of bark, berries, leaves, and roots, first pulverize them into a powder in a spice mill or coffee grinder, then take the powdered mixture in a capsule or teaspoon or pour boiling water over it and let it steep before drinking.

Make liver-supporting herbs a regular part of your liver-friendly regimen. It's especially important to take a combination of liver herbs whenever you feel sluggish, have overindulged with food or drink, or feel achy, depressed, or fatigued. Anise, fennel seed, ginger, licorice root, and peppermint make infusions (teas) that are pleasant to taste and soothing to digest. Use one of them as a flavor enhancer along with three or four bitter herbs. These herbs are available at most natural food stores and can be made into a tea. Don't add sweetener; just drink the tea straight like the medicine it is. Herbs that help the liver are almost always bitter; that's why they're effective for detoxification. Taking them with an aromatic herb will help the medicine go down more easily.

Medicinal plant juices are also available at natural food stores. Those that specifically support the liver include black radish juice, dandelion juice, and nettle juice. Artichoke is a member of the thistle family and a natural liver tonic; it stimulates the production and flow of bile and aids the detoxi-fication process.

Bitter Herbs and Taste Enhancers

Pair any of the bitter herbs in the left column with some of the flavorful herbs and spices in the right column.

	anise (*Pimpinella anisum*)
	catnip (*Nepeta cataria*)
barberry (*Berberis vulgaris*)	cayenne (*Capsicum frutescens*)
goldenseal (*Hydrastis canadensis*)	fennel seed (*Foeniculum vulgare*)
milk thistle (*Silybum marianum*)	ginger (*Zingiber officinale*)
skullcap (*Scutellaria lateriflora*)	gravel root (*Eutrochium purpureum*)
walnut bark (*Juglans nigra*)	licorice root (*Glycyrrhiza glabra*)
wormwood (*Artemisia absinthium*)	lobelia (*Lobelia inflata*)
	marshmallow root (*Althea officinalis*)
	peppermint (*Mentha piperita*)
	rue (*Ruta graveolens*)
	wild yam (*Dioscorea villosa*)

Culinary Herbs

The use of herbs in cooking has grown in popularity now that home chefs are aware of the wonderful qualities of these common plants. Culinary herbs are not only the oldest but also among the most popular taste enhancers, since they come from nature's bounty and not from the chemist's laboratory. Fresh herbs are always best to use, and they are now readily available, even throughout winter. There's a nutritional as well as flavor benefit from the vital life force of the fresh plant compared to the dried herbs that have sat on spice racks for years.

The custom in East Indian households is to put herb seeds, such as anise, dill, and caraway, on the dining table to chew during or after meals as a digestive aid. Peppermint is also soothing to both the stomach and digestive tract.

Use herbs generously and creatively when preparing your meals. Fresh herbs will keep for a few weeks in the refrigerator when wrapped in a damp paper towel and then placed in plastic wrap or a storage container. In addition to tasting delicious, herbs contribute to overall well-being and promote a healthy liver.

The following are a few harmonious vegetable-and-herb combinations that will support your liver and help you season your dishes to perfection:

- beets: basil, bay leaf, cardamom, dill, marjoram, oregano, tarragon
- Brussels sprouts: basil, caraway, dill, savory, thyme
- cabbage: caraway, celery seed, dill, summer savory, tarragon
- carrots: basil, dill, marjoram, parsley, thyme
- cauliflower: dill, rosemary, summer savory, tarragon
- cucumber: basil, savory, tarragon
- green beans: basil, dill, oregano, rosemary, thyme
- onions: basil, oregano, thyme
- peas: basil, dill, mint, oregano
- potatoes: basil, chives, dill, marjoram, mint, parsley
- spinach: oregano, rosemary, tarragon
- squash: basil, dill, oregano, savory
- tomatoes: basil, bay leaf, oregano, parsley

Planning the Liver-Cleansing Menu

For most people, planning healthy meals requires a firm rein on ingrained habits. Write down your particular dietary goals. It will be easier to stick to them when you read them over every day.

Fresh Vegetable Juice

A healthy liver is the result of a regular diet of nutrient-dense foods. Vegetables help to both cleanse and build the liver. In the form of freshly pressed vegetable juice, they're easy to digest and quickly deliver a nutritious punch of vitamins and minerals to the body. Drink at least eight ounces of freshly pressed juice daily. You should actually "chew" the vegetable juice in order to stimulate the salivary glands and start the digestive process. The more regularly you include vegetable juice in your diet, the easier it will be for your liver to function normally.

Beets, cabbage, carrots, celery, cucumbers, and spinach are all easy to juice and can be used in various combinations. My favorite mix is apple, carrot, and celery juice with a little ginger for extra flavor and its liver-loving properties. But since I consider freshly pressed juice medicine as well as food, I include some bitter greens: dandelion leaves, endive, and radicchio. Radish, especially black radish, with its sharp, biting edge, is also an excellent liver stimulant. I also make a point of adding beets to my juice regularly. They're an ideal blood cleanser.

I mention a compatible combination in the recipe section to get you started if juicing is new to you, but you can create your own combinations according to what you like, what's available, and what will facilitate the cleansing process. Cabbage, lettuce, radish, and spinach are all juiceable. Wild greens, such as dandelion, lamb's quarters, and pigweed, are available to many people; use them as long as you're sure they haven't been sprayed with pesticides.

Juicing three times a day is recommended if you have the time. You can flash chill your juice to preserve its freshness for one to two days. Put bottles of fresh juice in the freezer until the juice is about 40 degrees F, but be sure not to let it freeze. Using an infrared thermometer makes it easy to check. You can make your juicing regimen fit your lifestyle, but it's better to adjust your lifestyle to fit what's best for your liver.

Breakfast

Your body has properly fasted since the last meal at six o'clock the previous day. Your liver has been able to complete its task of detoxification during the night, and you wake refreshed. You practically bounce out of bed! The nourishment the liver likes at this point is the juice of half a lemon in a glass of distilled water, followed by two to three more glasses of water and maybe a cup of liver-cleansing tea—without sweetener. Then take a brisk walk for an hour, or perhaps spend half an hour on the exercise machine and half an hour jogging. In the summer, weed the garden; in the winter, spend an hour in the local pool or at the gym. I prefer walking in the fresh air all year long, no matter what the weather. By this time you've earned your first meal. Make it light. Have your fresh vegetable juice now or have a fresh grapefruit or other fruit, with more fruit midmorning. If you need something more substantial, this is a good time to enjoy a dish of muesli or cooked brown rice cereal, buckwheat cereal, millet cereal, or oatmeal. Take a digestive enzyme when you eat cooked food.

Muesli

Muesli is an uncooked breakfast food made with grains and fruit, traditionally soaked oat flakes and grated apple. It's been popular with many Europeans for decades and is now a staple in North America. If you make your own muesli rather than buying it packaged from the supermarket, you will have more control over the ingredients and can include your favorites while avoiding any added sugar.

You don't have to eat muesli just for breakfast, however. It's a wholesome snack any time of day; it could even be tucked into a lunchbox for a midday treat. Follow my suggestions for making homemade muesli with the recipe for Bircher Muesli with Sesame Seeds (page 35), or create your own version with oats, chopped nuts, berries, peaches, and grated apple. Add lemon juice and nut milk to moisten.

Midday Meal

When you're at home, you're able to prepare this most important meal. When you're at work, you'll probably have to prepare your lunch in advance and carry it with you. Take fresh ingredients for a salad, along with cooked grains and a few toppings or condiments. The noon meal should be unhurried and relaxed. Avoid eating a quick, light lunch so you don't stuff yourself at the dinner table and then go to bed with a full stomach.

Main Dishes

For most people, the evening is reserved for the main meal of the day, as it's a time when all the family is home and can cook and share food together. Be sure to accompany your main dish with a salad of raw greens or grated root vegetables. Remember that at least 75 percent of your diet should consist of raw (uncooked) foods.

A Healthy Liver for Life

Adhere to the liver-cleansing diet for a minimum of twenty-one days or longer, preferably for a full three months. It may take that long for you to fully experience the maximum benefits. Afterward, you may feel so fit that you'll want to stay on it for the rest of your life. Once your liver has released its toxic burden, the improvements to your health will be obvious and no longer will you feel sluggish. Your liver will be able to handle an occasional indulgence, but only as long as liver cleansing becomes a way of life.

Recipes

Bircher Muesli with Sesame Seeds

Makes 2 servings

Treat yourself to this gourmet muesli, but remember to eat it slowly, savor
the flavor, and chew it thoroughly so you'll be able to assimilate all the nutrients. Sesame seeds are rich in calcium and other minerals as well as unsatu-
rated fats. They've been widely consumed for thousands of years in China,
Ethiopia, India, and Mexico. Opt for seeds that haven't been roasted, since
heat damages the seed's oil. Freshly ground flaxseeds are another delicious,
high-quality ingredient to add to muesli, so take your pick.

⅓ cup rolled oats

1 teaspoon raisins

½ cup nondairy yogurt

3 tablespoons wheat germ

2 tablespoons pure maple syrup

2 bananas

4 teaspoons raw sesame seeds or freshly ground flaxseeds

Put the oats and raisins in a small bowl. Cover with lukewarm water and let soak
for at least 10 minutes or up to 12 hours. Drain. Add the yogurt, wheat germ,
and maple syrup. Thinly slice the bananas, add to the mixture, and stir until well
combined. Sprinkle the seeds over the top of the muesli just before serving.

Tofu and Salad Greens

Makes 2 servings

I love eating fresh, firm tofu when it's been cubed and marinated in tamari. This recipe makes a substantial meal, especially if you treat yourself to a second helping. Experiment by combining different oils to make the dressing.

Marinade and Tofu

¼ cup tamari

2 teaspoons toasted sesame oil

1 teaspoon lemon juice

Pinch cayenne

1 pound firm organic tofu, cubed

Dressing

¼ cup cold-pressed oil (such as flaxseed, olive, safflower, sesame, or
   sunflower oil)

Juice of ½ lemon

Dash tamari

Pinch cayenne

Salad

2 tomatoes, chopped

2 stalks celery, chopped

2 green onions, chopped

10 edible pea pods, sliced

6 mushrooms, sliced

6 florets cauliflower, blanched in hot water for 2 minutes

¾ cup alfalfa sprouts, lightly packed

Mixed organic salad greens

Ruby-red grapefruit segments

To make the marinade, put the tamari, oil, lemon juice, and cayenne in a medium bowl and stir to combine. Add the tofu and stir gently until evenly coated. Cover and let marinate in the refrigerator for 2 to 12 hours.

To make the dressing, put the oil, lemon juice, tamari, and cayenne in a small jar. Seal tightly and shake well to combine.

To make the salad, put the tomatoes, celery, green onions, pea pods, mushrooms, cauliflower, and sprouts in a large bowl. Add the tofu and dressing and toss gently until evenly distributed. Serve on a bed of salad greens with grapefruit segments on the side.

Colorful Cabbage Salad

Makes 2 servings

Cabbage is one of the most versatile vegetables. It tastes great cooked or raw and is rich in vitamins and minerals. Enjoy this eye-catching salad all year long.

Dressing

½ cup cold-pressed walnut, hazelnut, or flaxseed oil

1 tablespoon cider vinegar

Juice of one lemon

Freshly ground anise seeds

Dill seeds

Veggies

½ small green cabbage, julienned (about 2 cups)

½ small red cabbage, julienned (about 2 cups)

½ red pepper, julienned

½ yellow pepper, julienned

½ red onion, julienned

½ cup fresh, raw corn kernels

½ cup chopped fresh pineapple

Finely chopped fresh parsley

Finely chopped fresh mint

2 large cabbage leaves

Red and yellow pepper strips

To make the dressing, put the oil, vinegar, and lemon juice in a small jar. Season with anise seeds and dill seeds to taste. Seal the jar tightly and shake until the dressing is well combined.

To prepare the veggies, blanch the julienned green and red cabbage in boiling water for 30 seconds. Transfer to a large bowl and add the julienned red and yellow pepper, onion, corn, and pineapple. Add the dressing and toss gently to combine. Add parsley and mint to taste and toss again gently until evenly distributed. Serve in a cabbage-leaf cup garnished with strips of red and yellow pepper.

Waldorf Salad

Makes 2 servings

This traditional Waldorf salad is abundant in calcium, iron, magnesium, potassium, and vitamins B, C, and E. Celeriac, also known as celery root, is especially good for the liver. If you don't have any on hand, celery can be used instead.

½ cup almonds, soaked in water for 8 to 12 hours

⅔ cup water, plus more as needed

½ cup plain nondairy yogurt or vegan mayonnaise

1 tablespoon lemon juice

2 tablespoons raisins, soaked in water for at least 10 minutes
    or up to 12 hours

1 cup peeled and julienned celeriac or sliced celery

2 apples, cubed

¼ cup chopped raw walnuts or cashews

2 large leaves butter lettuce

Watercress, for garnish

Drain the almonds and transfer them to a blender. Add the water and process into a thick cream. Add 1 to 2 tablespoons of additional water if needed to facilitate processing or achieve the desired consistency. Transfer to a medium bowl. Add the yogurt and lemon juice and stir until well combined.

Drain the raisins and add them to the bowl along with the celeriac, apples, and walnuts. Stir until well combined. Put one of the lettuce leaves on a plate and top with half the salad. Repeat with the remaining lettuce leaf and salad. Garnish each serving with watercress.

Ratatouille

Makes 2 servings

Serve this cooked dish with steamed brown rice, millet, or potatoes, accompanied by a salad of raw greens or grated root vegetables. That's a complete meal!

2 tablespoons extra-virgin olive oil

1 red onion, finely chopped

4 cloves garlic, minced

2 carrots, cut into 1-inch pieces

3 stalks celery, cut into 1-inch pieces

1 eggplant, cut into 1-inch pieces

1 yellow pepper, cut into 1-inch pieces

1 red pepper, cut into 1-inch pieces

2 small zucchini, cut into 1-inch pieces

4 beefsteak tomatoes, cut into 1-inch pieces

1 teaspoon tomato paste

1 sprig fresh marjoram, or ⅛ teaspoon dried

1 sprig fresh sage, or ⅛ teaspoon dried

1 sprig fresh tarragon, or ⅛ teaspoon dried

1 sprig fresh thyme, or ⅛ teaspoon dried

1 bay leaf

½ teaspoon ground turmeric

Pinch sea salt

Chopped fresh parsley, for garnish

Heat the oil in a large skillet or wok over low heat. Add the onion and garlic and cook, stirring frequently, for 3 minutes. Add the carrots and cook, stirring frequently, for 5 minutes. Add the celery and cook, stirring frequently, for 5 minutes. Add the eggplant, yellow pepper, and red pepper and cook, stirring frequently, for 5 minutes. Add the zucchini and tomatoes and cook until the tomatoes just begin to soften, about 3 minutes. Add the tomato paste, marjoram, sage, tarragon, thyme, bay leaf, turmeric, and salt and stir until evenly distributed. Cook, stirring occasionally, for 10 to 30 minutes, until hot and the flavors have married. Remove the bay leaf and sprinkle with parsley just before serving.

Pumpkin-Broccoli Pot

Makes 2 servings

This wonderfully warming dish will satisfy two hungry people when served with cooked millet or buckwheat.

1½ teaspoons extra-virgin olive oil

1 cup peeled and cubed pumpkin

2 cups chopped broccoli

2 tablespoons water

1 tablespoon lemon juice

½ teaspoon dried dill weed

Sea salt

Freshly ground pepper

¼ cup plain nondairy yogurt (optional)

Put the oil in a large saucepan and heat over low heat. Add the pumpkin and cook, stirring frequently, for 4 minutes. Add the broccoli, water, lemon juice, and dill weed and cook, stirring frequently, until the broccoli is tender but still bright green, 4 to 5 minutes. Don't overcook. Season with salt and pepper to taste. Stir in the optional yogurt just before serving.

Tomato-Broccoli Simmer

Makes 2 servings

This dish is hearty enough to eat on its own, but I like it best served over rice or quinoa. Putting a little water in the pan before you heat the olive oil will prevent the oil from getting too hot. Sometimes I eliminate the oil and just cook the veggies in water.

1 tablespoon extra-virgin olive oil

1 small shallot, minced

2 cloves garlic, minced

2 cups chopped broccoli florets and stems

1 teaspoon lemon juice

Pinch cayenne

Chopped fresh basil

Chopped fresh oregano

1 cup chopped tomatoes

10 pitted black olives, sliced

Put the oil in a large saucepan and heat over low heat. Add the shallot and garlic and cook, stirring frequently, for 2 minutes. Add the broccoli, lemon juice, and cayenne and stir to combine. Add as much fresh basil and oregano as you like and stir until evenly distributed. Cover and cook for 5 minutes. Add the tomatoes and cook, stirring occasionally, just until all the vegetables are tender, 2 to 3 minutes. Stir in the olives and serve.

Rhody's Health Combo

Makes 1 serving

This tasty, liver-cleansing vegetable juice combines antioxidant-rich root vegetables and greens.

3 carrots

1 beet

3 or 4 leaves dandelion

1 or 2 large stalks celery

1 (1-inch) cube ginger

Juice all the ingredients according to the manufacturer's directions for your juicer. Serve immediately.

Aunt Rhody's Seedy Soup-and-Salad Topping

Makes as much as you like

I've been making this nut-and-seed topping for years. I like to sprinkle it on salads, soups, and vegetables. Use a coffee grinder or spice mill to grind the seeds. Seeds taste best when they're freshly ground, so don't make too large a quantity at once.

Nutritional yeast powder or flakes

Powdered psyllium husks

Chia seeds, freshly ground

Flaxseeds, freshly ground

Sunflower seeds, freshly ground

Fennel seeds, freshly ground

Sesame seeds, lightly toasted in a dry cast-iron skillet

Use equal amounts of each ingredient or according to your taste. Put all the ingredients in a bowl and stir until well combined. Store in a glass jar or airtight container in the freezer to prevent the essential fatty acids in the flaxseeds from becoming rancid.

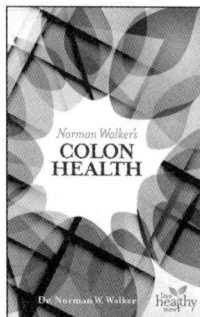

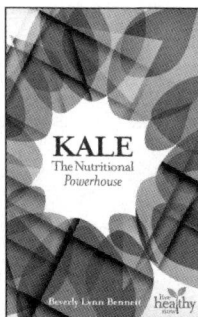

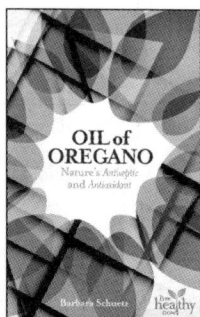

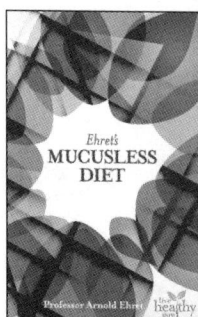